An Herbal Sampler

A Notebook for Women

Edited by
Elaine Goldman Gill

Designed by
Jane Twentyman MacDonald

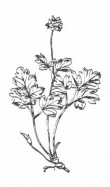

THE CROSSING PRESS/TRUMANSBURG, NEW YORK 14886

Printed in the U.S.A.
Typesetting by Martha Jean Waters

ISBN 0-89594-146-5
Copyright © 1984 The Crossing Press

Introduction

I have found several herbals helpful, but the herbalist I respect most is Juliette de Baraicli Levy whose advice seems to me most grounded in experience with animals, people and her own children. She is also familiar with the medicines of nomadic people, Arabs and gypsies, and thus draws from other, older cultures. Moreover, she seems to be a true healer, with humility and love for people. I would advise anyone interested in herbs to go directly to her books. A short bibliography appears at the end of this sampler.

I have respect for herbs as medicines found in nature, not manufactured in a laboratory. However, I urge all readers not to assume that because herbs are natural, they are harmless. Some of the herbs described here are quite powerful. In all cases, I would like people to err on the side of caution and, when trying an herb for the first time, to take little and observe their reactions carefully. There are variations in response to an herb, just as there are to penicillin.

The advice of a good herbalist is beyond price. Self help can go only so far—for a complex diagnosis and prescription, seek someone professional.

I would also like to make a case here for a very simple remedy—raw food. Raw food detoxifies the body. I believe at least fifty percent of the food we eat should be raw and, if there is something seriously wrong with us, that percentage should be increased.

If raw foods have too much fiber to be tolerated by the body, they can be juiced. There are several types of juicers on the market. In many European spas the juice of vegetables and fruits is regularly given to patients. These juices are referred to as the blood of the plant, life-giving forces.

I also would like to promote the use of lemons and limes as wonderful astringents to tone the body. Dr. Luelle Hamilton, my doctor, and others urge the use of half a lemon or one lime squeezed into a glass of warm water as the first food of the day. Baraicli Levy states she has cured many animals and people with lemons. I can believe it because I have seen the effect of these fruits on my own body.

The best way to take herbs is to eat them raw. Dried, they may be made into a tea. Herbalists recommend different procedures, either adding the herb to boiling water or vice versa. I don't really see the difference. I do think it best not to have the herb come into contact with metal. I use glass or enameled saucepans or bowls, wooden spoons and bamboo strainers. Let the herb steep for six to twelve hours, covered. When the tea is poured off into a jar, do not cover the jar with a lid. Baraicli Levy advises using a cotton square secured with a string or rubber band. The standard proportion is one tablespoon of the dried herb to one pint of water. Baraicli Levy gives another method for making an infusion. Put one cup of shredded fresh herbs in a shallow glass dish filled with water and expose to direct sunlight for forty-eight hours.

There is much help in nature for us if we would but look and try.

E.G.G.

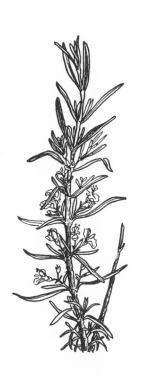

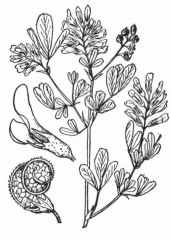
Alfalfa

Henry Bieler recommends alfalfa to alkalize sick bodies rapidly. Since sick people tend to be acidic, the alfalfa brings them into balance, detoxifying the liver in the process. Use the dried or fresh leaves steeped in boiling water as tea.

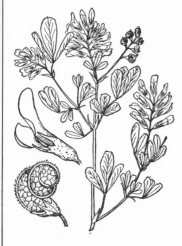

Alfalfa

Alfalfa sprouts are wonderful in salads, adding crunch, vitamins and minerals; they are particularly welcome in winter when good fresh greens are not easily come by.

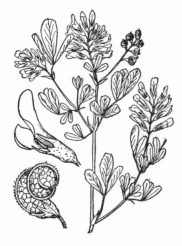

Alfalfa

Alfalfa is reputed to be helpful for teeth. I am not sure this is true; I do know that six months after I stopped taking alfalfa tablets, my teeth, which had been trouble-free for several years, began to decay.

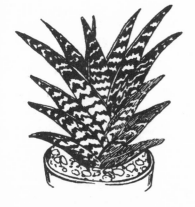

Aloe

Aloe is the common house plant. Keep it on a window near the kitchen stove. When you inadvertently burn yourself, pluck the healthiest spike from the plant, squeeze from the cut end, and apply to the burned skin. It also eases poison ivy rash. Baraicli Levy says she uses banana peels, applying the inside surface to the burned area.

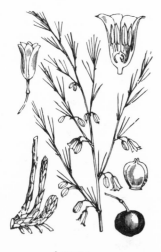

Asparagus

Asparagus is one of the very best kidney cleansers. In early spring, it's a wonderful treat to munch a handful of raw stalks. Or saute them lightly so they stay crunchy. Or juice them raw or frozen. If you don't have enough asparagus, add some raw celery juice.

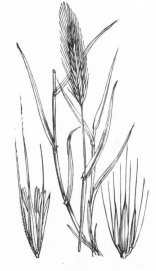

Barley

I used barley gruel to help my year-old son who had severe diarrhea over a long period of time. Boil the barley until it is soft and force it through a sieve. Most children and adults will like the taste.

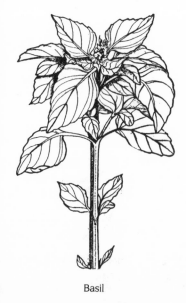

Basil

Basil has a long history as a sacred herb. According to Mrs. Grieve, "Every good Hindu goes to his rest with a basil leaf on his bosom as his passport to paradise." As a tea, it eases indigestion.

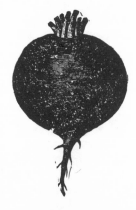

Beets

Beets are a good liver detoxifier. Since beets are very powerful, take in very small doses, either grated raw or juiced in the raw state. I mix ten parts raw apple juice to one part raw beet juice.

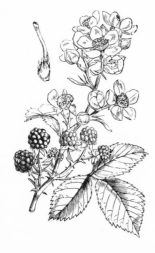

Blackberries

Blackberries strengthen the blood and are therefore good for anemia. It is best to eat them raw or crush them in a blender and force through a strainer. Dilute with water and sweeten with a bit of honey if you wish.

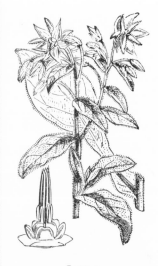

Borage

Arab women chew raw borage leaves to increase their milk supply.

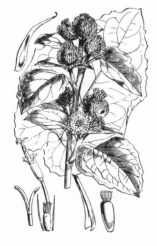

Burdock

Burdock root is valued in macrobiotic cooking, sauteed or used in soups. It is sweet tasting, reminiscent of parsnips. It is also a good kidney cleanser. It is claimed that all parts of burdock (leaves, roots, seeds, flowers) are medicinal. It's nice to know that burdock, the most obnoxious weed in a garden, is good for something.

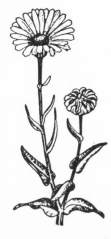
Calendula

Calendula, or pot marigold flowers, can be dried, crushed and mixed with cold cream for a healing salve, good for chapped, rough skin.

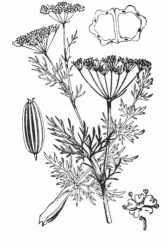

Caraway

Caraway seeds are excellent for digestion. Chew a few before meals or steep them in boiling water and drink as tea.

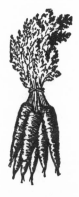

Carrots

The ordinary garden carrot is very high in vitamin A which many of us need badly. It's best to juice the carrots raw and drink a small glass as a tonic. Baraicli Levy claims that carrots are rich in insulin and are therefore excellent food for diabetics.

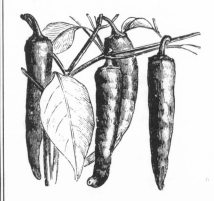

Cayenne Peppers

Mexicans say that if visitors eat salsa, their pepper sauce, they won't get *la turista*. Cayenne fights bacteria internally.

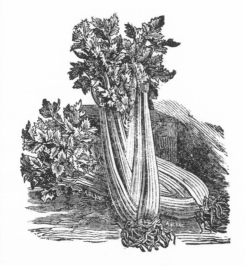

Celery

Celery is high in sodium and therefore is a natural tonic. Juice the raw stalks for a very refreshing drink.

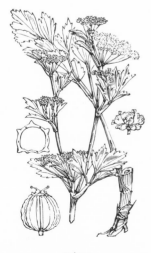

Celery

Celery seed is also medicinal. Keep a shaker filled with the seeds on the table and sprinkle freely on salads.

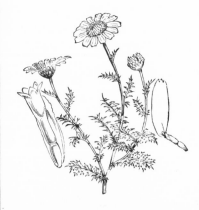

Chamomile

Chamomile flowers can be steeped in boiling water, cooled and used as a hair rinse, particularly good for blondes who wish to lighten their hair.

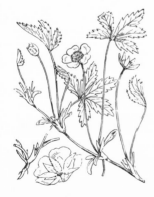

Cinquefoil

The Latin name for cinquefoil is *potentilla reptans, potentilla* meaning powerful. Baraicli Levy claims the herb is very valuable as an astringent. She recommends syringing a diffusion of the leaves into the nostrils to cure sinus infections.

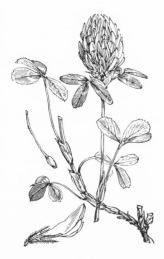

Red Clover

Red clover, like alfalfa, alkalizes the body. It's easiest to take clover as tea: cover the dried flowers with boiling water and steep.

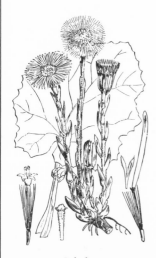

Coltsfoot

Coltsfoot soothes irritated mucus membranes. A tea made of the leaves will help expel mucus from throat and lungs.

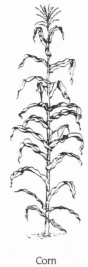

Corn

Corn silk, the fine strands that surround the cob, that you fastidiously pick off before you boil it, can be steeped, either fresh or dried, as a tea to reduce a swollen prostate gland.

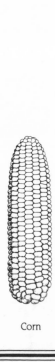

Corn

Modern nutritionists claim that corn is not a nutritious grain in that it doesn't supply complete protein. However, I have observed that cats and dogs are crazy for anything that has corn in it. According to Baraicli Levy, "Corn is the only known cereal which alone can sustain man without any other food over a long period." I believe it.

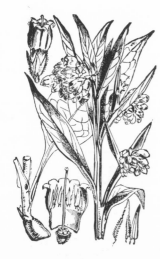
Comfrey

Comfrey is king of the garden, surviving and thriving almost anywhere with little or no care. According to most herbalists, this is a wonder plant, good for whatever ails you. I have come across one warning, urging pregnant women to be careful using it.

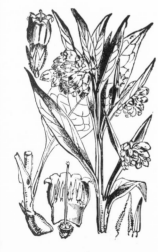

Comfrey

Shred a few comfrey leaves in salad. Put a half leaf into you cup to brew with alfalfa tea. A poultice of the macerated leaves is supposed to be excellent for bruises.

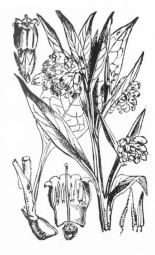
Comfrey

Comfrey root is also medicinal. Clean and cut in small pieces, cover with boiling water and drink for chest ailments.

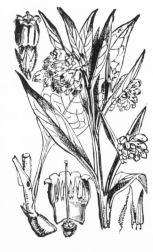
Comfrey

Comfrey was called knitbone by country people and used for this purpose before modern bone setting techniques. It is still good, Baraicli Levy claims, for strained or weak ligaments and muscles, rheumatism or arthritis.

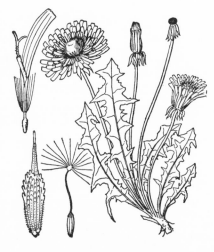

Dandelion

Shred the young dandelion leaves into salads along with other greens for a good blood cleanser. A section of the root can be cut up fine and swallowed for kidney and bladder problems.

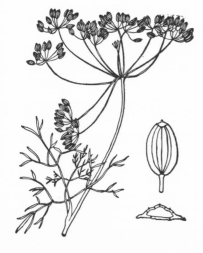

Dill

A mild dill tea (made from the seeds and water) is recommended by some herbalists for infants a few minutes before they begin to breastfeed to improve their digestion.

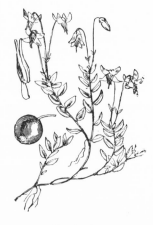

Cranberries

Cranberry juice is a good kidney cleanser; it can help clean up a bladder in-
fection.

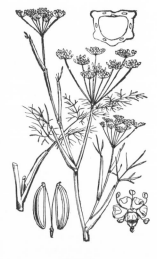
Fennel

Arabs use the fennel root, grated fine and mixed with bran as a laxative before meals two times a day. Fennel seed is supposed to cut appetite.

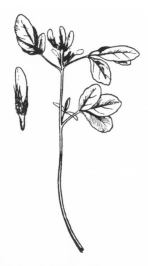

Fenugreek

Fenugreek seeds, like flax seeds, yield much mucilage when soaked in water. Eat the soaked seeds to quiet inflamed mucus membranes throughout the body.

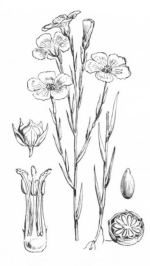

Flax

A teaspoon of flax seed can be swallowed dry or first soaked until it becomes a glutinous mass and then swallowed. Either way, the seeds gently scrub out and clean the intestines.

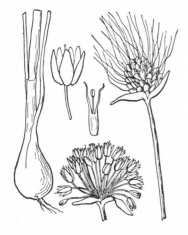

Garlic

A Mexican healer I know put garlic cloves on an Indian woman's gangrenous foot and cured her. Garlic is a powerful anti-bacterial agent, used either externally or internally. The same healer claims that eating fresh garlic several days before going abroad can prevent travellers' diarrhea.

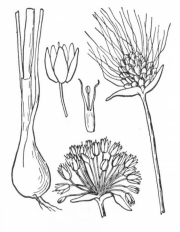

Garlic

If you use garlic medicinally or simply like the taste and don't want to offend your neighbors, chew some parsley afterwards. The Mexican healer I mentioned earlier carries a clove or two of garlic in his pocket and chews whenever he feels like it. He, like many herbalists, thinks it's a cure-all.

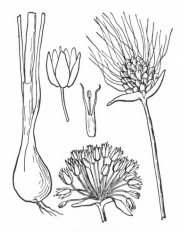

Garlic

Garlic provides a gentle stimulus to the digestive tract. It is best eaten raw, crushed in a mortar and pestle and put into salad dressing or combined with the liquids of a salad dressing in a blender and pulverized.

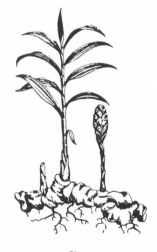

Ginger

The Chinese value ginger as a blood warmer and digestive aid. Chew on a bit of the raw root or use it grated fine in stir fries. I keep it covered in the refrigerator in a plastic bag to prevent it from drying out. When I saute chopped garlic for a stir fry, I grate some ginger root directly into the wok.

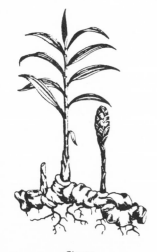

Ginger

The Chinese not only like the effects of ginger on the system—they like the taste. Chinese restaurants keep grated raw ginger covered with peanut oil in jars in the refrigerator, ready for quick frying.

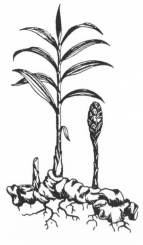

Ginger

Grated ginger root steeped in boiling water and made into a hot tea is supposed to bring on delayed menstruation.

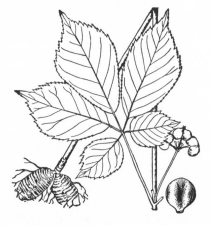

Ginseng

Ginseng is prized by Asiatic people as a restorative. Taken as tea, it relieves fatigue and gives energy. The Chinese use it for men only, but I know several women who use ginseng regularly and value it.

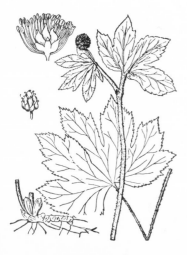

Golden Seal

The root of golden seal is a powerful antibiotic, much esteemed by Native Americans who used it as a cure-all. It is particularly helpful in ridding the body of excess mucus. The dried root is powdered and generally swallowed in capsules—the taste is very bitter. I find this herb very strong and urge caution in using it.

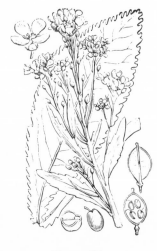

Horseradish

My doctor, Dr. Luelle Hamilton, claims that grated raw horseradish expels excess mucus. Clean and peel finely a section of the root, grate it and cover with fresh lemon juice. Kept tightly covered in the refrigerator, it is good for about ten days. Take a teaspoon with fruit or vegetable juice two times a day.

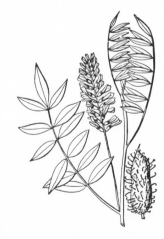

Licorice

Licorice root contains cortisone, good for chest ailments. Put the shredded root into boiling water and steep. Most people like the sweet taste of this tea.

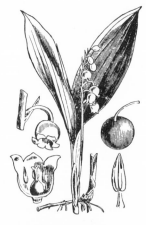

Lily Of The Valley

Baraicli Levy claims lily of the valley flowers are medicinal, providing a good heart tonic. Take two handfuls of the flower spikes, cover with 1 1/2 pints of boiling water and drink as tea.

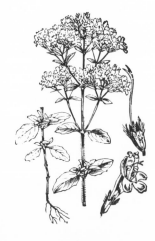

Marjoram

Marjoram is good for digestion. Sprinkle the raw leaves in salads or use the dried leaves for tea.

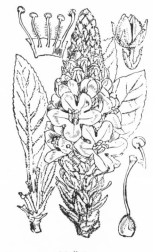

Mullein

I can personally testify that hot mullein tea (made from dried, crushed leaves in boiling water) helps asthma by loosening packed mucus in the lungs. I used a cup two times a day. It is particularly good at night when asthmatics suffer most.

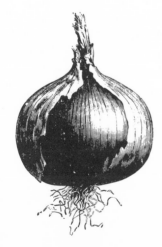

Onions

Onions are reputed good for the urinary tract. Grate an onion finely and put into salads. Use plentifully in soups, stir fries and stews.

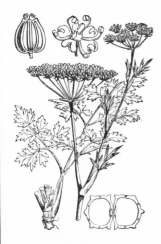

Parsley

Make a lotion of parsley leaves, seeds and water and rub into the scalp to foster healthy hair. Parsley is also reputed good for gall bladder troubles.

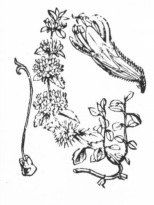

Pennyroyal

Pennyroyal is a flea killer, sprinkled on cats and dogs and rubbed into the skin. I have several people's remedies to offer for fleas. Dr. Luelle Hamilton recommends bathing an afflicted cat with a coconut shampoo (a foaming shampoo), drying it and then sprinkling brewers yeast plentifully all over the cat, rubbing it in thoroughly. Then she advises wrapping the animal in a towel, scratching its ears to keep it quiet and waiting until the fleas suffocate.

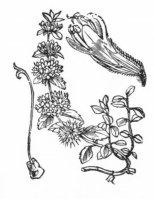

Pennyroyal

The novelist, Marge Piercy, on the other hand, uses a very fine steel comb for her cats. Each time she withdraws the comb from the animal's fur, she thrusts the comb into a pot of boiling water to kill fleas and flea eggs. She repeats this process at intervals to keep the animals free of fleas.

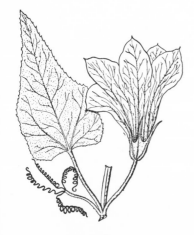

Pumpkin

Baraicli Levy claims that the flowers, fruits and seeds of pumpkin are all medicinal: the flowers make a tonic tea; the fruits, grated raw, strengthen the blood; the seeds expel tape worm.

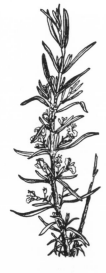

Rosemary

Like comfrey, rosemary is a cure-all herb much prized by herbalists. Baraicli Levy recommends it particularly for all female ailments, including threatened miscarriage.

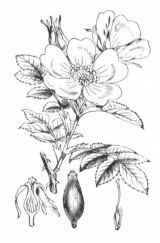

Roses

Rosehips, the fruits of roses, make an excellent tea, full of vitamins and
reputedly good for all female ailments.

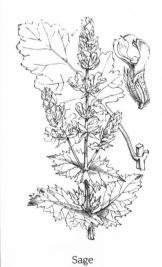

Sage

Ben Harris recommends hot sage tea as a gargle for sore throat. He says it will flush excess mucus from the bronchial tubes.

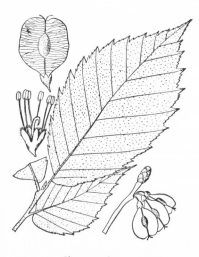

Slippery Elm

The bark of slippery elm is valuable for soothing swollen mucus membranes anywhere in the body. Make a paste with warm water and take a spoonful at a time or drink as tea.

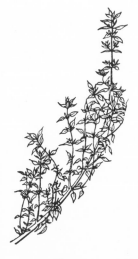

Thyme

Hot thyme tea is good for chest ailments. Arabs make a mixture of dried powdered thyme, roasted sesame seeds and coriander seeds (ground fine) and salt. They eat this with olive oil on bread. Sounds wonderful.

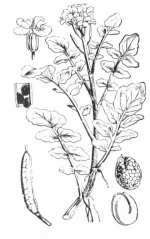

Watercress

Ben Harris claims that watercress is vitamin rich and will strengthen the bloodstream and is also a good remedy for skin disorders. Eat the leaves and stems in salads.

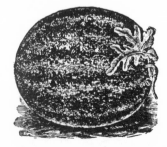

Watermelon

I put watermelon pulp into a blender and strain out the seeds and fiber. The juice is a very good kidney cleanser. I recommend drinking it a few days before the onset of menstruation.

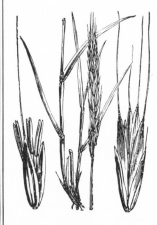

Wheat

Wheat bran is good for making food move down the digestive tract faster and keeping the body efficient. Some folks I know keep bran in a sugar bowl on the table and spoon it over granola, yogurt or hot cereal.

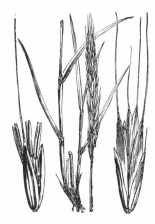

Wheat

Wheat germ is an extraordinary food, the heart of the wheat loaded with vitalizing Vitamin E. But be careful the germ is not rancid when you buy it. Smell it—it should be sweet. And when you take it home, keep it tightly covered in a glass jar in the refrigerator and use it quickly.

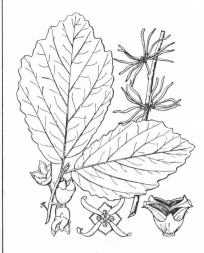
Witch Hazel

Witch hazel is a good astringent. Applied externally, it heals bruises and wounds.

Helpful Books

Henry Bieler, *Food Is Your Best Medicine*, Keats Publishing

Juliette de Bairacli Levy
  Common Herbs for Natural Health, Schocken Books
  Herbal Handbook for Farm and Stable, Rodale Press
  Nature's Children: A Guide To Organic Foods And Herbal Remedies for Children, Schocken Books

Mrs. M. Grieve, *A Modern Herbal*, 2 vols., Dover Press

Ben Charles Harris, *The Compleat Herbal*, Barre Publishers, Barre, NH